Quick & Easy way to LOOK BEAUTIFUL
THE NATURAL WAY

Nita Mehta

B.Sc. (Home Science), M.Sc. (Food and Nutrition), Gold Medalist

SNAB Publishers Pvt Ltd

Quick & Easy way to
LOOK BEAUTIFUL
THE NATURAL WAY

© Copyright 1996-2005 **SNAB** Publishers Pvt Ltd

WORLD RIGHTS RESERVED. The contents—all recipes, photographs and drawings are original and copyrighted. No portion of this book shall be reproduced, stored in a retrieval system or transmitted by any means, electronic, mechanical, photocopying, recording or otherwise, without the written permission of the publishers.

While every precaution is taken in the preparation of this book, the publisher and the author assume no responsibility for errors or omissions. Neither is any liability assumed for damages resulting from the use of information contained herein.

TRADEMARKS ACKNOWLEDGED. Trademarks used, if any, are acknowledged as trademarks of their respective owners. These are used as reference only and no trademark infringement is intended upon.

9th Print 2005
ISBN 81-86004-14-9

Food Styling and Photography: **SNAB**

Layout and laser typesetting :

National Information Technology Academy
3A/3, Asaf Ali Road
New Delhi-110002
☎ 23252948

Published by :

SNAB
Publishers Pvt. Ltd.
3A/3 Asaf Ali Road,
New Delhi - 110002
Tel: 23252948, 23250091
Telefax: 91-11-23250091

Editorial and Marketing office:
E-159, Greater Kailash-II, N.Delhi-48
Fax: 91-11-29225218, 29229558
Tel: 91-11-29214011, 29218727, 29218574
E-Mail: nitamehta@email.com
snab@snabindia.com
Website: http://www.nitamehta.com
Website: http://www.snabindia.com

Distributed by :

THE VARIETY BOOK DEPOT
A.V.G. Bhavan, M 3 Con Circus,
New Delhi - 110 001
Tel : 23417175, 23412567; Fax : 23415335
Email: varietybookdepot@rediffmail.com

Printed by :
BRIJBASI ART PRESS LTD.

Rs. 89/-

Dedicated to my Father
Late Shri Harbans Lal

Foreword

Women have always desired to look beautiful. Beauty is the outcome of **constant care**. Many young girls, just before their marriage, suddenly want their skin to turn petal soft, their hair to turn shiny & lustrous and start looking beautiful. Unfortunately, there is no magic wand which can do so. Not only this, but also no amount of make-up can camouflage the flaws on the skin caused by indifference & neglect. Making yourself beautiful is not difficult, if you make the beauty care fit into your daily routine. Just 10-15 minutes of daily beauty care with easily available, inexpensive ingredients from the kitchen shelf will make you feel confident & proud of yourself. So make beauty care a **habit**, just as brushing your teeth!

A balanced diet is very important for the skin and hair. Fresh fruit juices & salads should be a part of your daily menu. So **diets & habits** are important in beauty care. So, here's all you need to look good & feel great!

Nita Mehta

Contents

Fresh Faces 9

    Know your skin   10
    Daily skin care   11
    Practical tips & home made recipes   13
    Your weekly programme through nature   15
    'Fairer you'   19
    Special masks for different skins   20
    The right way to massage   25
    Black heads   28
    Ageing problems   31
    Anti-wrinkle masks   33
    Skin polishers   36

Tanned skin in winters 38
Banishing pimples 39
Party face-tighteners 40
Rose water after bath body lotion 41

Sparkling Teeth 42

Bright Eyes 43
Tired aching eyes 44
Sparkling eyes 45
Puffiness in eyes 47
Massage around the eyes 48
Dark circles 51
Scanty eyebrows 52

Lustrous Hair 55
- Herbal Shampoo 55
- Dull, lifeless hair 56
- Dandruff 57
- Henna 62,63

Pretty Hands 64
- Hand lotion 66

Soft Feet 69

Your Wardrobe 73
- A Short female 74

    A plump female 75

Balanced Diet 76
    Slimming tips 77
    Tomato juice 78
    Carrot & guava juice 79
    Vitamin C booster 80
    Strawberry delight 81
    Health Tip 82

Beautify Your Soul 83

Fresh Faces

The face care extends to the neck. Use a flat face brush to apply the pastes & move the brush in the upward direction while doing so. The secret of a healthy, glowing complexion is a sound skin care routine & a diet rich in vitamin A & C.

Know Your Skin

It is always easier to look after your skin if you are sure about the type of skin you have.

Normal : The skin is smooth, finely textured, soft & supple.

Dry : The skin is usually thin and delicate, often flaky, and prone to fine lines.

Oily : The skin is shiny and coarsely textured, often with enlarged pores and prone to blackheads and spots.

Combination : This skin consists of both dry and oily areas. The fore head, nose & the chin are oily forming a 'T' shape of oily area on the face. The cheeks & temples (just above the end of the eye brows) are dry.

Daily Skin Care

Cleansing, toning, moisturising are the fundamental routine which should be followed for a glowing complexion. You may do it at night before going to bed. If you have an oily skin you should follow this routine in the morning too.

Cleansing : Wash your face with a good face wash. Do not wipe by rubbing the skin. Simply **pat dry**. For thorough cleansing, dip a piece of cotton wool in 1 tbsp milk. The milk should be unboiled preferably. Squeeze it gently. Rub on the face & neck in a circular, upward motion to **deep cleanse** your skin. This opens the pores of the skin & cleanses it thoroughly. Cleansing should continue until there are no traces of dirt on the cotton wool.

Toning : As cleansing opens pores, it is important to use an astringent to close them. An astringent also freshens your face besides closing the pores. Instead of a ready-made astringent, just splash chilled water on your face & then pat dry with a towel. Chilled water or preferably cold mineral water is an excellent astringent & skin freshener which tones your face well. Toning also removes the last traces of dirt.

Moisturising : A moisturiser will replace natural oils lost through cleansing and toning, keeping your skin supple and protecting it against moisture loss. Use a herbal moisturizing lotion or a night cream. Lightly massage onto the skin using **circular up & outward movements.**

Practical Tips
&
Home made Recipes for a
Glowing Complexion

Every morning, start the day with
a glass of warm water
juice of ½ lemon

1 tsp honey
mixed together
It helps to clear digestion & hence your skin glows.

Drink 8 glasses of water each day for a
radiant skin.

Your weekly programme through Nature

Do it at any time of the day. Remember to clean your face first.

Monday...
Scrub a piece of cucumber on your face & neck. Wash off with cold water after 15 minutes.

Tuesday...
Rub half a tomato on your face & neck. Rinse off after 15-20 minutes.

Wednesday...
Scrub a piece of lemon. Rinse off after 15-20 minutes.

Rub in an upward & circular motion.
Repeat for the next three days of the week.

Weekend Routine

Sunday.....

Pamper your face with an almond-honey mask

Mix

4-5 almonds (soaked & skin removed) - ground to a fine paste

½ tsp honey

1 tsp milk - enough to make a paste

Apply on your face & neck. Wash off after 15 minutes.

If you are always in a hurry, grind ½ cup almonds with their skin to a powder & bottle it. Make a paste of 1 tbsp almond powder mixed with 1 tsp honey & enough milk.

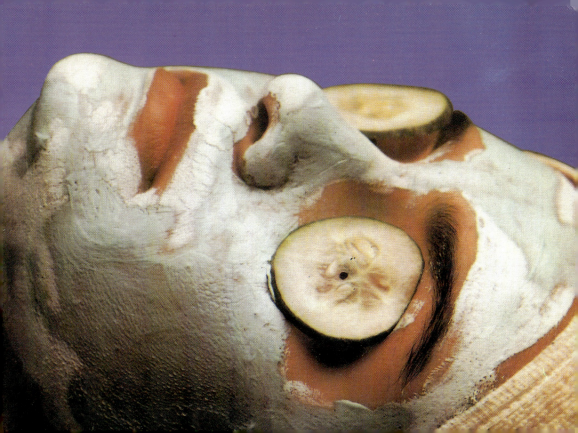

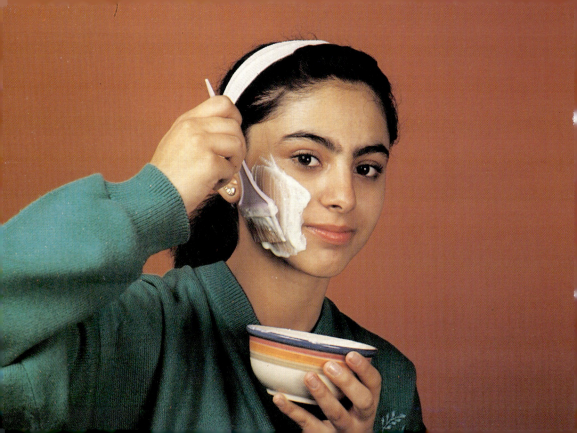

"Fairer You"

For a fairer, clearer complexion use a whitening lotion every day.

Mix

1 tbsp cucumber juice (grate 1" piece of unpeeled cucumber & squeeze through a muslin cloth)
few drops lemon juice
a pinch of haldi (turmeric) powder

Dampen a piece of cotton wool & squeeze it. Dip in the above lotion. Rub it all over the face & neck. Keep for ½ hour. Wash off with water.

Special Masks for Different Skins

Understand your type of skin by reading on page 10 and unmask your beauty by deciding on the right face mask.

Apply the mask atleast once a week with a flat face brush, moving the brush in the upward direction.

A face mask helps to draw out dirt from clogged pores. It gives a smooth complexion to the user.

Multani Mitti with Rose Water for Oily Skin

Mix to form a paste
1 tbsp multani mitti (fuller's earth)
rose water - enough to make a paste

1. Apply the paste on the face and neck.
2. Rinse off after 10-15 minutes.

Egg & Honey Mask for Oily Skin

Mix
1 tsp honey
½ tbsp of egg white

1. Break an egg & separate the white. Take out ½ tbsp of egg white in a small bowl. Keep the rest in the fridge (or use it up for breakfast!)

2. Mix honey & apply on the face & neck with a brush.

3. Rinse after 7-10 minutes.

Potato Yoghurt Mask for Dry Skin

Mix

1 tbsp finely grated raw potato

1 tsp thick curd

1. Wash & cut a small potato. Grate finely. Press the grated potato to extract the juice. Mix curd.

2. Apply on face & neck with a brush. Move the brush in the upward direction.

3. Leave for 15 minutes. Wash off.

Olive Oil & Malai Mask for Dry Skin

Mix
1 tsp olive oil or almond oil
2 tsp fresh malai

1. Apply on face with a brush. Massage for 2 minutes in the upward direction with the fingers so that it gets absorbed. Leave for 10 minutes.

2. Wash with warm water. Remove excess with cotton wool pads soaked in warm water.

3. Splash cold water on the face. Pat dry.

The Right Way to Massage
Sketches on page 26

A wrong massage can prepone wrinkles & a right massage can postpone wrinkles. So, do it the right way!

To Massage....

1. Start at the collar bone and brush fingers up neck and under chin. Roll knuckles over cheeks and gently roll skin between fingers until it tingles. See sketch 1.

2. Position thumbs under chin and starting at the inner

The Right Way to Massage

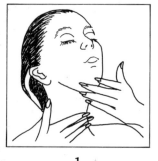

1

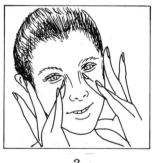

2

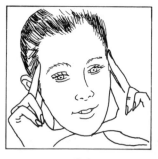

3

corners of eyes run fourth finger gently over brow bone and down below eyes into corners again. Massage with a **very light touch.** Sketch 2.

3. Place first and second fingers on temples and rotate firmly, without moving fingers, pressing as you go. Finish with a firm stroke towards the centre of the fore head. Massage the forehead upwards with the fingers of both the hands alternately. Sketch 3.

Black Heads

Black-heads are caused by over active oil producing glands (sebaceous glands) of the skin. The excess secretion of oil expands and thickens the pores of the skin. The oil collects in the pores and hardens into a plug. The pores are then clogged with hardened sebum or oil. Since the pores are open, the tip of the clogged grease is exposed to the air and oxidizes, turning black. Hence, the name black-heads.

Washing the face twice a day with a medicated soap and lukewarm water helps reduce the oiliness of the skin surface and eliminates the chances of black-heads.

For Removing Blackheads..

Mix in a large pan

5-6 cups water, juice of 1 lemon

1. Keep the pan on fire to boil.
2. Rub cold cream on the black-heads.
3. Keep a large towel ready.
4. Remove the pan of boiling water from fire.
5. Bend over the steaming hot water & cover your head with the towel.
6. Steam for 10 minutes.
7. Rub the black-heads vigorously with a face towel.
8. Wash with chilled water. Repeat twice a week.

Grandmother's Tips for Black Heads

To avoid black heads...

Mix

1 tbsp husk obtained by sifting wheat flour (chokkar)
1 tsp milk (enough to form a thick, dry paste)

Sift chakki ka atta of ordinary quality to get the husk. Make a very thick paste with milk & rub it on the black heads on your nose for 1-2 minutes daily. You may rub the left over on your face too.

For removing black heads.....

Mix 1 **tsp mitha soda (soda-bicarb)** in 2-3 drops water to make a thick paste. Rub on your nose on the black heads.

Ageing Problems

A mature woman can look young in her late forties if wrinkles are postponed with the right care during her youth.

Protect yourself from the **harsh rays** of the **sun**. Invest in a pair of good quality sun glasses to avoid getting wrinkles at the outer corner of the eyes (crow's feet). Your eyes tend to shrivel up in the sun & wrinkles come at the outer corners of the eyes.

Try to be relaxed & tension free. Overlook small, petty matters. Have a sound 8 hour sleep. Massage your face in the right way (p 27) to postpone wrinkles. Follow the daily beauty care routine as given on page 11 to look young.

Tips for Preventing & Curing Wrinkles

- Massage your face & neck with **almond oil** (Badaam rogan) with upward, circular motion. The oil is available even with chemists.
- Cut a **vitamin E capsule open**. Mix Vitamin E capsule (opened up) & enough glycerine to make a paste. Apply on your face with a brush in the upward direction. Wash off after 10-15 minutes.
- **Fresh malai** (not for oily skins) left on the face overnight, is very effective for wrinkles.
- An effective, simple exercise to keep your facial muscles tight. Fill your mouth with air as if you are filling air into a balloon. Keeping the air trapped in the mouth, carry it to the side into the cheek, thus **blowing your cheek**. Now rotate the air to the other cheek. Repeat it several times. You can feel the muscles being pulled. Do it any time - reading a book, driving a car ……

Anti Wrinkle Masks

Mix

½ tbsp cornflour & ½ tbsp honey

1. Make a paste together without any lumps.
2. Apply on the face & let it dry. Rinse off after it dries.

OR

Mix

1 tsp malai, 2 tbsp egg white

1. Beat eggwhite. Add malai & mix to form a paste.
2. Apply on the face & neck for 20 minutes. Rinse off with warm water.

Honey-Carrot Anti Wrinkle Mask

Mix

1 tbsp honey

1 tsp carrot juice (grate a small piece of carrot & squeeze through a muslin cloth)

1. Apply on the face & neck.
2. Keep cucumber slices on your eyes & relax for 20 minutes.
3. Add a pinch of soda bicarb in ½ cup warm water.
4. Dip cotton wool in this warm water & remove the mask with it.

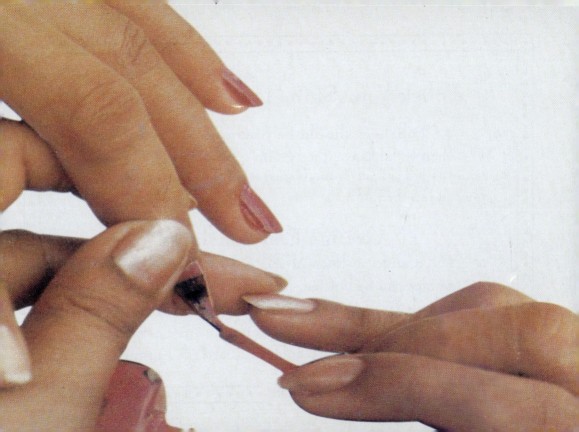

Polish Your Skin 'The Natural Way'

Polishers should be used once a week.

The slightly, abrasive tiny grains present in the polishers, remove the dead cells from the surface of the skin, leaving a fresh smooth face behind.

Orange Peel Polisher

- The orange peels are **dried & powdered finely**. The powder can be bottled. Mix 1 tbsp powder with enough unboiled milk to make a thick paste. Massage by rubbing it gently on your face with an upward, circular motion for 1 minute. Rinse with cold water after 5-7 minutes.

Maize Polisher

- Wash face. Do not wipe. Take 2 **tsp makki ka atta** on your palm and rub it on your **wet face** for a few seconds. Wash off.

Husk Polisher

- **Sift** ordinary quality chakki ka atta to get the **husk**. Mix **1 tbsp husk (bran)** of atta (wheat flour) with a few drops of **rose water**. Apply on your face. Massage gently on your face with an upward, circular motion for 1 minute. Rinse with cold water.

Tanned Skin in Winters

In winters , bleach the tanned skin with walnut or vinegar.

Mix to form a paste

1 walnut - powdered (can be done on a chakla-belan)
1 tbsp milk, few drops rose water

Cover face & neck with the paste. After it dries, rub it upwards. Wash off.

OR

Mix

1 tsp honey with a few drops of vinegar

Apply on your face & neck for 15 minutes. Wash off.

Banishing Pimples

Pimples arise due to internal problems. Have a well balanced diet, rich in vitamin A. Keep the stomach clean by drinking 8 glasses of water daily. Avoid oily, masale wala khaana & aerated drinks. Keep the face clean by always washing it with a medicated soap whenever you come from outside. Do not rub your face to wipe. Just pat dry.

- Grind mint (poodina) leaves. Apply generously & allow to dry. Wash off.

OR

- Mix together 1 tbsp besan (gram flour), ½ tsp haldi (turmeric powder), 1 tsp lemon juice & enough milk to make a paste. Apply on your face for 20 min. Wash off.

Party Face-Tighteners

Here are face-tighteners to brighten your face before going to a party. Beat one **egg white** and apply on your face with a brush. After it dries up (15-20 min), wash off with warm water. Splash cold water on the face. Pat dry.

Make a paste of 1 **tsp cornflour**, 1 **tsp wheat husk** (obtained after sifting ordinary quality wheat flour) & enough **malai** to form a thick paste. Rub on your face & neck. Rinse after it dries. The corn starch tightens the skin, the husk removes the dead cells & the malai provides the nourishment.

Rose Water After Bath Body Lotion

This after-bath lotion will replace the natural oils lost through bathing and will leave your skin feeling luxuriously smooth and soft.

125 ml rose water
1 tsp lemon juice
2 tsp honey
2 tbsp almond oil
4 drops oil of rose
100 ml glycerine

1. Warm rose water over low heat and stir in the lemon juice and honey until dissolved. Remove from heat, add almond oil, rose oil and glycerine. Beat the mixture until it emulsifies.
2. Store in a sterilized tightly capped bottle. Apply generously to the body after bathing, massaging well into the skin.

Sparkling Teeth

Rub teeth once a week with

lemon juice mixed with a little table salt

OR

table salt mixed with a few drops of mustard oil

OR

soda bicarb

Any of these will give a sparkle to your teeth.

Bright Eyes

Get plenty of sleep. Aim for 7-8 hours sleep each night. Avoid late nights.

Treat sleep like a bank. Put in extra hours when you have overdrawn.

For Tired Aching Eyes ...

Dip cotton wool pads in ¼ cup chilled milk. Squeeze gently. Place on closed eyes for 10 minutes. Listen to a soothing music.

Put cucumber slices on closed eyes for 10 - 15 minutes.

For Sparkling Eyes

Soak

1 tsp of **dried amla** in a cup of clean water at night.

Next morning, strain the water through a muslin cloth. Dilute the water by adding another cup of water & splash the eyes with this water.

It may hurt the eyes slightly but it's certainly very good for eyes.

It is essential to remove all
EYE MAKE-UP
at night.

Puffiness in Eyes

Rub a slice of raw potato gently on the area around the eyes.

OR

Grate a potato & tie it in a muslin cloth. Keep on the eyes.

This relieves puffiness & makes the eyes fresh & clear.

Massage Around The Eyes
Sketch on page 49

Always massage with a **light, feathery** touch.

While massaging the skin around the eyes, start from the **outer** corner of your eye, move **below** your eye using your fore finger.

As you reach near your **nose**, take a '**U**' turn and massage with an extremely light touch **over** the upper lid towards the outer corner of the eye or the starting point.

Massage both the eyes with fingers of both the hands simultaneously.

Massage Around The Eyes

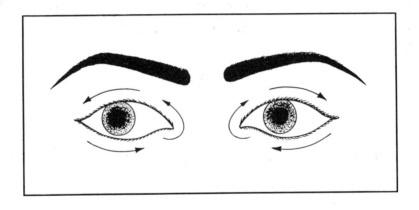

Do not stretch or rub the **delicate skin around the eyes** when applying any cream or lotion on your face. Any massage around the eyes should be done with a very **light & a feathery** touch.

Avoid the **area around the eyes when you apply face masks** as the skin around the eyes is very delicate.

Dark Circles

Lack of sleep may be a cause for the dark circles under your eyes. Have enough sleep & a diet rich in fresh fruits & uncooked vegetables.

Apply **juice of cucumber** on the dark circles every day with a damp piece of cotton. To take out cucumber juice, grate a 1" piece of unpeeled cucumber and squeeze through a muslin cloth.

OR

Mix 1 tsp **tomato pulp grated on the grater**, a pinch of **haldi** (turmeric pd.), ½ tsp **lemon juice** & 1 tsp **besan** (gram flour) together to form a paste. Apply with a brush on the dark circles every day. Wash off when it dries.

Scanty Eyebrows

Make your eyebrows thick & shiny by applying castor oil on them.

Whenever you oil your hair, remember to rub oil on the eyebrows also.

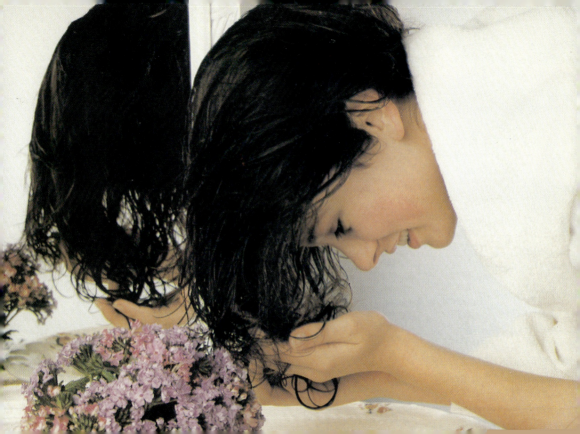

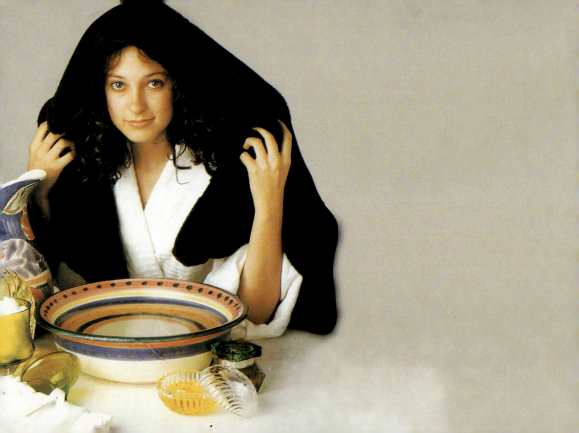

Lustrous Hair

Herbal Shampoo

2 reethas (break to remove seeds)
2 shikakai pods
2 tbsp dried amla

1. Mix all ingredients together with 2 cups of water in a pan at night. Boil in the morning till it is reduced to half.
2. Remove from fire & cool. Mash the herbs well.
3. Strain through a plastic soup strainer. Use this water as a shampoo on wet hair.

There will be no lather but the hair will certainly get cleaned.

A listless hair massage with oil is useless..

1. While massaging, place the fingers **firmly** on the head.
2. Work in small **circular strokes**, first clockwise & then anti-clockwise, moving the skin of the scalp as you do so. It is **not your fingers** but the skin of the **scalp that should move**.
3. By massaging this way, the **blood circulation** to the scalp is improved which keeps your hair strong & healthy.

For Dry, Lifeless Hair...

1. Rub a little warm olive oil or coconut oil right into the roots of the hair by dividing the hair into sections.

2. Soak a towel in steaming hot water and squeeze & wrap it around the scalp for 10-15 minutes. This opens up the pores of the scalp.

3. Give a second massage to the hair (without oil) for better & deeper absorption of oil.

4. Wash off after 1 hour.

If you opt for ready made shampoos..

Egg shampoos are good for

DRY OR NORMAL hair.

For OILY HAIR, use a

lemon based shampoo.

Brushing Your Hair

100 strokes a day is a myth!

Too much brushing is not good for oily hair because it stimulates oil glands that are already over active. So, do not brush too much if you have oily hair.

For dry hair, **correct** brushing is important. Sometimes dryness of the scalp is due to improper brushing. The brush bristles must be first **pressed gently into the scalp**, and then carried gently down to the hair tips. If the hair is brushed superficially, the oil glands become lazy because you are not exercising them sufficiently & your hair remains dry.

For Dull, Lifeless Hair

1. Soak 1 tbsp **methi dana (fenugreek seeds)** in a little water. Grind to a paste.
2. Rub it into your scalp. Leave for ½ hour.
3. Shampoo the hair as usual.

Whey Hair Rinse
rich in proteins to lubricate & strengthen hair.

Whenever you make **paneer** at home, collect the whey (greenish liquid). Strain & store in a bottle. Rub in the scalp on wet hair. Rinse with fresh water.

Dandruff

Dandruff can cause skin problems like pimples, acne or rash. Those prone to dandruff often have pimples on the forehead or cheeks or back. Keep the hair always clean. Applying thick curd on the hair & washing off with a good shampoo after ½ hour also helps.

To remove dandruff, do this once a week..

1. Oil the hair first with warm coconut or olive oil at night.
2. Next morning mix lemon juice with a little salt.
3. Rub it in the scalp with the empty peel turned inside out.
4. Leave for 1 hour. Wash hair as usual.

Henna as a conditioner for giving bounce & body to limp hair.....

Mix **henna powder** with some **lemon juice**. Add enough **curd** to form a thin paste. Apply on the hair, dividing it into sections. Shampoo after ½ hr. This is **not for colouring the hair.**

For giving a shine to the hair....

Give a final rinse to the hair after your head bath with **juice of 1 lemon or a few drops of vinegar added to ¼ bucket of water.**

Colouring Hair with Henna (Mehandi)

Coffee or Kaththa (catechu) added to henna paste gives hair a richer brown colour, rather than a reddish tinge. Add a little ground sugar & lemon juice also to the paste. Make the paste with tea water.

Colouring Hair with Chemical dyes

If you have opted for dyeing your hair with the readymade dyes (chemical dyes) available in the market, remember to apply a little cream on your eyebrows. This prevents the dye from coming in contact with the hair of the eye brows, while washing, forming a thin film on them.

Pretty Hands

The hand care extends to the elbows. Remember to scrub them while taking a bath.

Apply a good herbal moisturising hand cream morning and night.

Smoothen your hands, by applying a little curd on them. Rub the hands for a minute together with curd on them, as if you are washing them. Wash off.

When you apply your face mask, pamper your hands also with a bit of the same mask. Your hands get clean, soft and smooth.

Hand Lotion

A nongreasy lotion which repairs the damage done by house work.

Mix

3 tbsp rose water
2 tbsp lemon juice
1 tbsp glycerine

1. Mix all together & store in a refrigerator.
2. Rub a little on your hands every night.

Once a week dip your hands in warm water to which a little shampoo is added. Add 1 tsp of olive oil & ½ tsp haldi (turmeric) powder to the water. Scrub your fingers & nails with a nail brush. Clean the edges of the nails by rubbing with a piece of lemon. Lemon has a mild bleaching effect where as haldi softens the skin. Wash your hands after 10 minutes & massage the hands with the hand lotion as given on page 66.

Keep a nail file in your hand bag. You could keep your nails in shape while commuting without wasting any time.

File in one direction always.

Push back your cuticles (the skin from where the nail starts) to give length to your nails.

Before applying nail polish, push cotton wool pads between the toes to avoid smudging.

Soft Feet

Feet Care...

The best exercise for the feet is walking barefoot, on the grass, if possible.

Creaming feet daily goes a long way towards keeping the skin soft & adds to foot beauty.

Cracked Feet turn Baby Soft

Morning routine...

Rub heels with a pumice stone daily while bathing. It removes the dead skin without hurting. Massage a good hand & body lotion. Remove excess with a tissue.

Bed time routine...

Before going to bed, soak feet in warm water to which a small sachet of shampoo has been added. Wash after 10 minutes. Mix a few drops of lemon juice with 1 tsp vaseline taken out on the palm of your hand. Rub this lemon-vaseline into the cracked heels till it gets absorbed. You may wipe off the excess with a tissue.

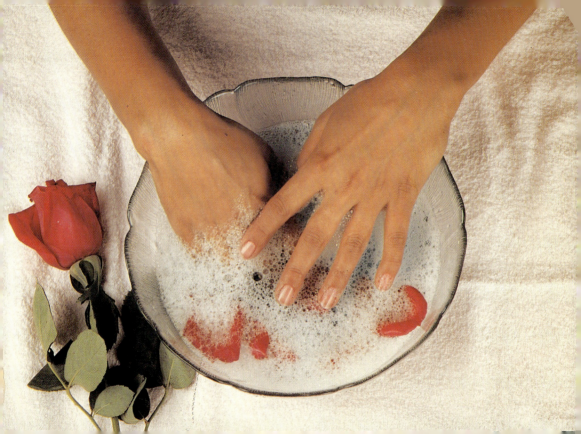

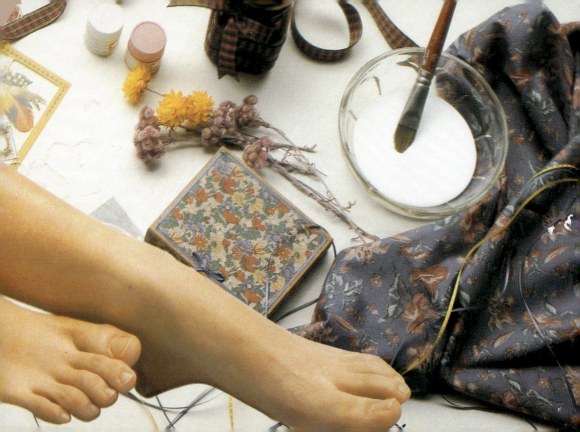

Your Wardrobe

Wear what suits you.
Do not follow fashions blindly.

A Short Female...

Avoid big prints, bold checks & stripes. These will make you look shorter. Fine stripes & checks, smaller prints will complement your stature.

Avoid buying sarees with broad borders. You may be tempted to buy them but remember they will only make you look even shorter. A small border will suit you better.

Horizontal stripes are not for you. Vertical lines will give you height.

A Plump Female...

Looks slimmer in dark shades. If black suits you, it is the ideal colour for you for a formal evening.

Do not wear big & bold prints.
Do not wear short tops. Longer tops will look better.

Balanced Diet

The condition of the skin & hair are dependent largely on the food you consume. Hence the importance of healthy, nutritive foods cannot be ignored. A protein rich diet is essential for the cell renewal process of the skin & hair. Include curd in your daily menu. Foods rich in Vitamin A like carrots & others rich in Vitamin C like tomatoes are excellent. Remember vitamin C gets destroyed on heating, so a fresh tomato juice is far more nutritive than a bowl of hot tomato soup.

Slimmers...

Slimmers should **not skip meals** in an effort to reduce. The number of meals should remain the same but the quantity at each meal should be reduced.

Eat a **plate of salad first** before you start your meal. Make salads a must with every meal, thus ensuring a big dose of vitamins for the whole family. Use whatever is in season - tomato chunks, carrot sticks or cucumber.

Eat slowly. Chew your food well. Do not swallow. Soon you will realize that the quantity of food consumed is less, yet more satisfying.

Tomato Juice

A quick healthy drink which improves your complexion.

1. Blend 4 ripe tomatoes with ½ cup of water in a mixer.
2. Mix in a pinch of salt & kala namak (rock salt). Add a tsp of sugar if desired.
3. Strain through a soup strainer. Add a little chopped poodina.

Carrot & Guava Juice

A drink rich in vitamins.

4 carrots - peeled
1 guava - washed

Juice carrots and guava in a juice extractor.
Add ice cubes if desired.

Vitamin C Booster

This juice supplies a real boost of vitamin C along with iron.
Vitamin C helps the absorption of iron.

3 oranges
1 apple - cored
juice of ½ lemon (optional)
salt & sugar to taste

Juice oranges and apple in a juice extractor. Add lemon juice & salt-sugar to taste. Pour over ice cubes.

Strawberry Delight

Treat yourself to this exotic tasting juice.

500 gm watermelon - skin and seeds removed
150 gm strawberries - hulled

Juice watermelon and strawberries in a juice extractor and pour over ice cubes.

Health Tip

To enhance the absorption of **iron** from cereals & vegetables, eat citrus fruits like oranges, rich in **vitamin C** immediately after meals.

Avoid consuming **tea & coffe after meals** as the tannins, present particularly in tea, reduce the absorption of iron

Beautify Your Soul

Each night before going to sleep, thank God for all He has given you.

A beautiful soul projects a beautiful appearance!

BEST SELLERS IN QUICK & EASY SERIES

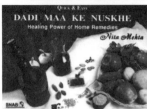
DADI MAA KE NUSKHE

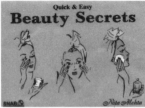
BEAUTY SECRETS

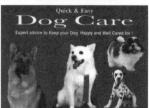
DOG CARE

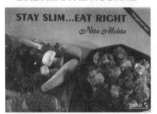
STAY SLIM...EAT RIGHT

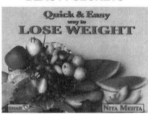
LOSE WEIGHT

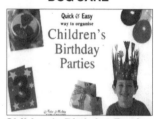
Children's Birthday Parties

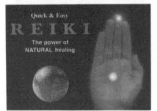
REIKI

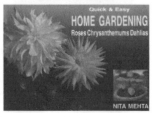
Roses, Chrysanthemums, Dahlias

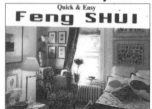
Feng Shui